Surviving History

THE PLAGUE

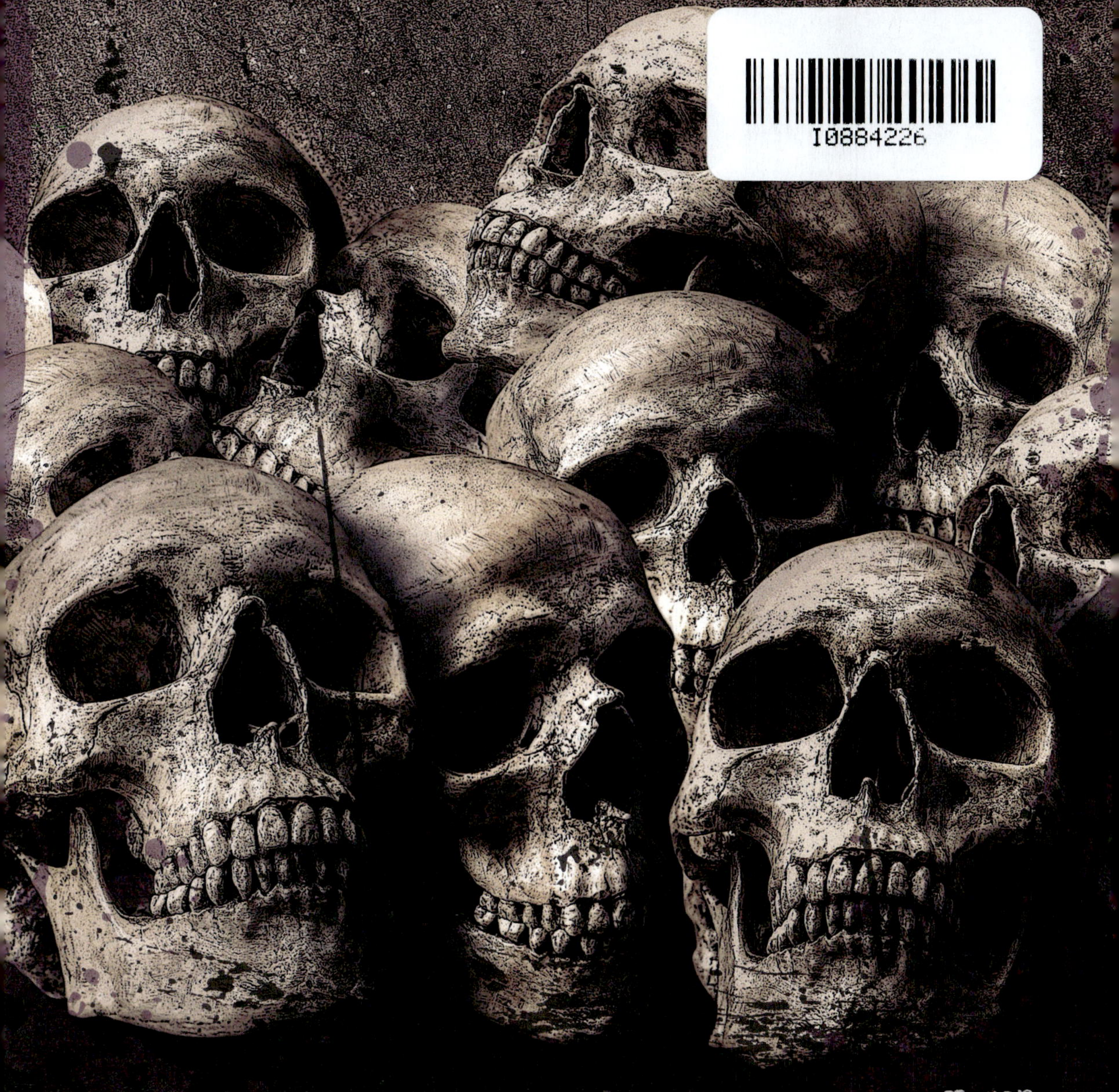

Virginia Loh-Hagan

45TH PARALLEL PRESS

Published in the United States of America by Cherry Lake Publishing Group
Ann Arbor, Michigan
www.cherrylakepublishing.com

Reading Adviser: Marla Conn, MS, Ed., Literacy specialist, Read-Ability, Inc.
Book Designer: Melinda Millward

Photo Credits: © Baimieng/Shutterstock.com, front cover, 1; © Erin Cadigan/Shutterstock.com, 4; © damianKuzdak/iStock.com, 6; © Daniel Samek/Shutterstock.com, 8; © Jarp2/Shutterstock.com, 10, back cover; © duncan1890/iStock.com, 12; © duncan1890/iStock.com, 14, 16; © Everett Collection/Shutterstock.com, 18, 24; © illustrissima/Adobe Stock, 20; © Morphart Creation/Shutterstock.com, 22; © ilbusca/iStock.com, 27; © Creative Images/Shutterstock.com, 28

Graphic Element Credits: © Milos Djapovic/Shutterstock.com, back cover, front cover; © cajoer/Shutterstock.com, back cover, front cover, multiple interior pages; © GUSAK OLENA/Shutterstock.com, back cover, multiple interior pages; © Miloje/Shutterstock.com, front cover; © Rtstudio/Shutterstock.com, multiple interior pages; © Konstantin Nikiteev/Dreamstime.com, 29

45TH Parallel Press is an imprint of Cherry Lake Publishing Group.

Library of Congress Cataloging-in-Publication Data

Names: Loh-Hagan, Virginia, author.
Title: The plague / by Virginia Loh-Hagan.
Description: Ann Arbor, Michigan : Cherry Lake Publishing, [2021] | Series: Surviving history | Includes index.
Identifiers: LCCN 2020030330 (print) | LCCN 2020030331 (ebook) | ISBN 9781534180277 (hardcover) | ISBN 9781534181984 (paperback) | ISBN 9781534181281 (pdf) | ISBN 9781534182998 (ebook)
Subjects: LCSH: Epidemics–History–Juvenile literature. | Communicable diseases–History–Juvenile literature. | Black Death–History–Juvenile literature.
Classification: LCC RA653.5 .L64 2021 (print) | LCC RA653.5 (ebook) | DDC 614.5/732–dc23
LC record available at https://lccn.loc.gov/2020030330
LC ebook record available at https://lccn.loc.gov/2020030331

Cherry Lake Publishing Group would like to acknowledge the work of the Partnership for 21st Century Learning, a Network of Battelle for Kids. Please visit http://www.battelleforkids.org/networks/p21 for more information.

Printed in the United States of America
Corporate Graphics

TABLE OF CONTENTS

INTRODUCTION

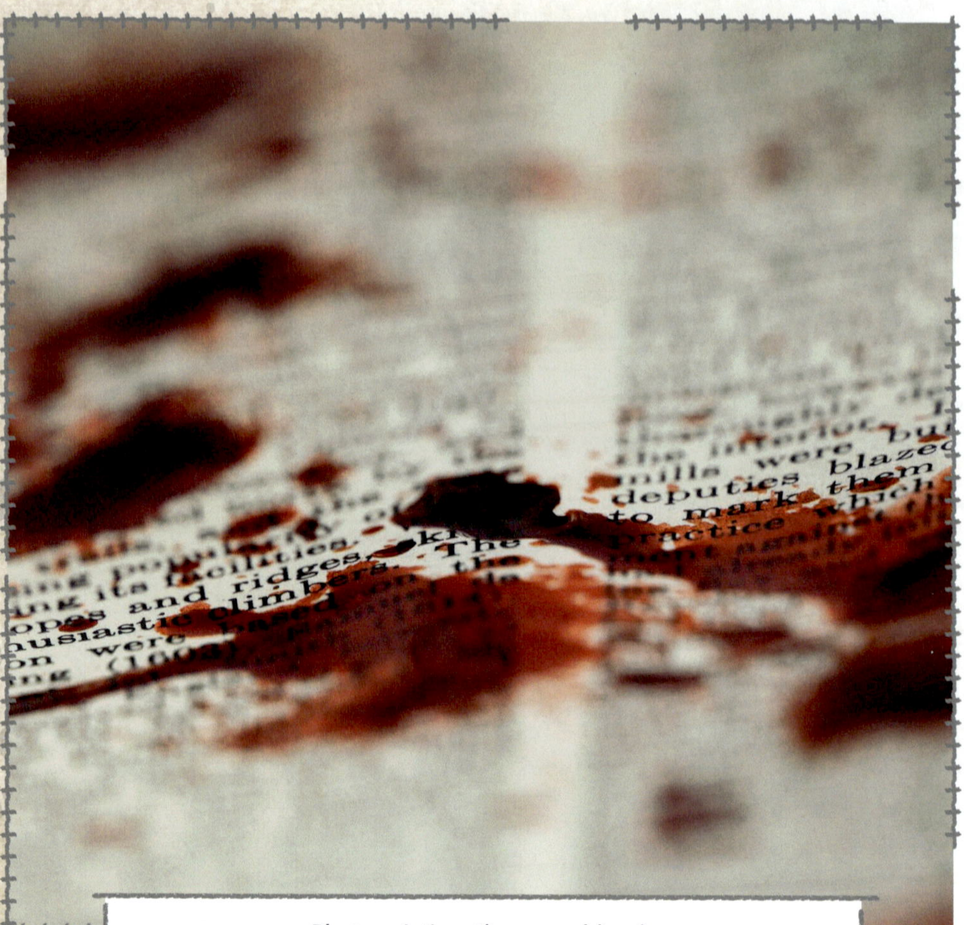

Plague victims threw up blood.

The **bubonic plague** was also called the Black Death. Bubonic refers to swollen glands. A plague happens when sickness spreads quickly. It kills a lot of people. The Black Death spread in Asia and Africa. It also happened in Europe. It happened in the 1340s to 1350s. It's the deadliest **pandemic** in human history. Pandemics are sicknesses that spread over a wide area.

Victims are people who suffer. Plague victims got fevers. They got aches and pains. They had **boils** on their skin. Boils are bubbles that form on skin. These boils oozed pus and blood. Some plague boils were as big as apples or eggs. Victims got red spots that turned black. These black spots meant the flesh was dead.

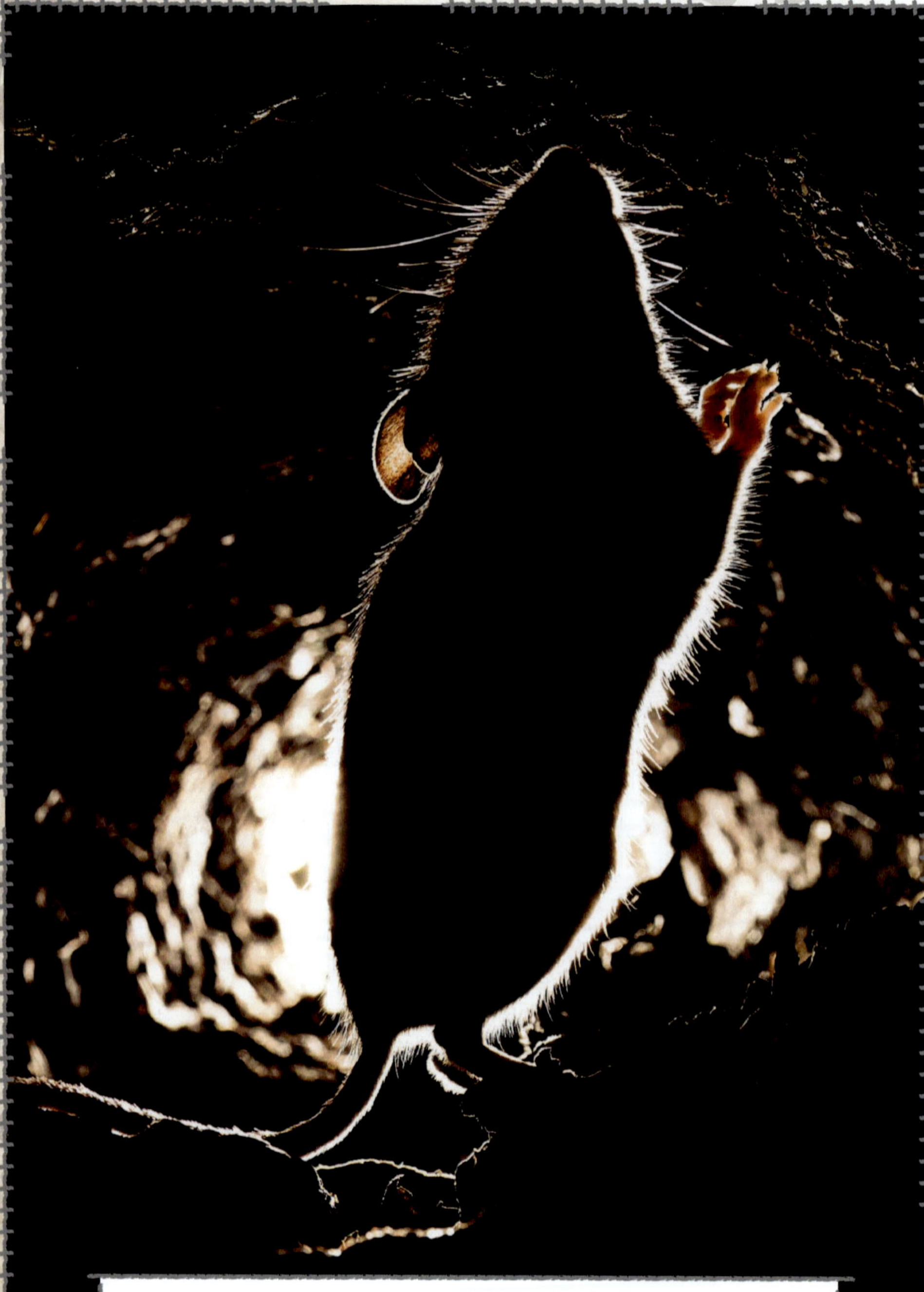

The plague was carried by fleas living on rats.

The plague started in Asia. It spread along the Silk Road. The Silk Road was a trade route. It connected Asia and Europe.

The plague attacked **medieval** Europe. Medieval means the Middle Ages. Fleas **infected** rats. Infect means to make sick. Rats and fleas bit humans. This spread the infection.

The plague spread through the dirty, crowded cities. Human and animal waste was in the streets. Water was **polluted**. Polluted means dirty. These conditions made the sickness spread more easily.

The plague slowed in the early 1350s. But it never really ended. It returned every 10 to 20 years.

SAFE OR AT-RISK?

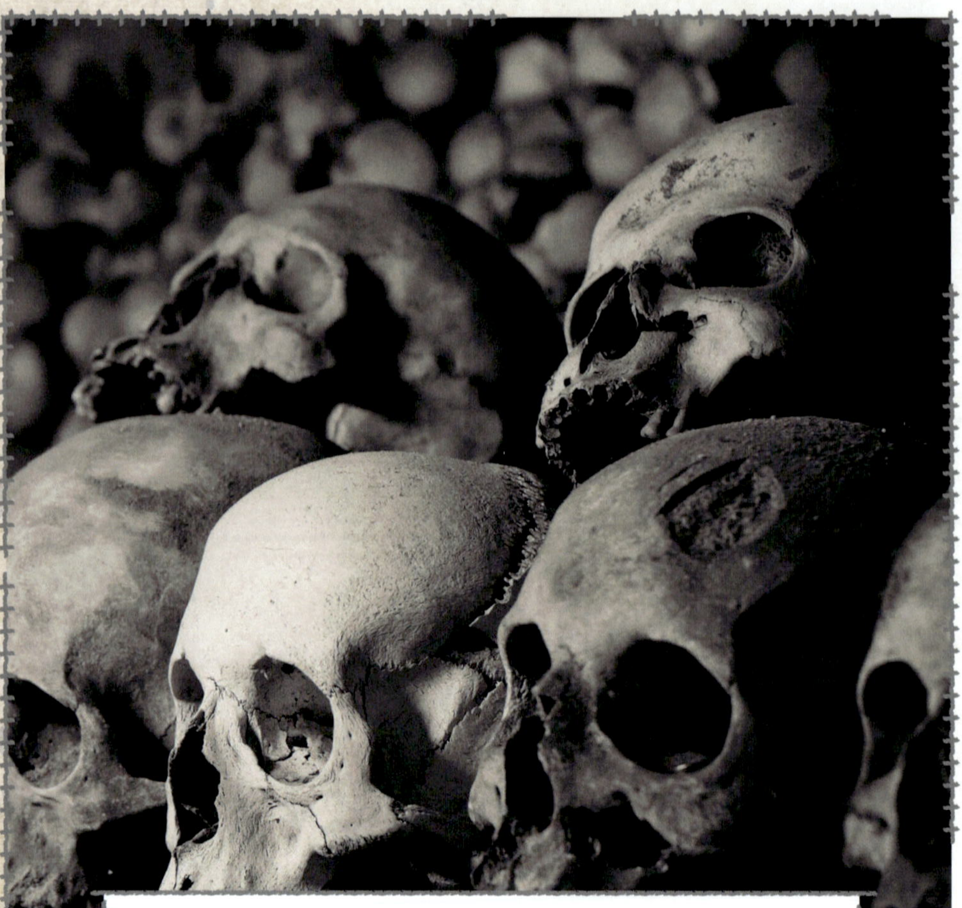

Ships carrying plague were called death ships.

The plague came to Europe in October 1347. Twelve ships arrived from the Black Sea. They docked at Messina. Messina is a port in Italy. Most of the sailors were dead. The other sailors were sick. They had black boils. Italian officials kicked the ships out. But it was too late. Infected ships had also arrived in other European cities.

Fleas and rats got ashore. They infected other animals. They infected humans. Plague germs survive a few days in rodents. They survive longer in fleas. When untreated, plague germs invade bloodstreams. They grow quickly. They attack the lungs. Once in the lungs, they could be **airborne**. Airborne means carried by air.

QUESTION 1

How likely were you to get infected with the plague?

A You were healthy before the plague came. You didn't have any sicknesses. Your body was strong enough to fight the plague.

B You were a young child. Or you were very old. You were already in poor health. You had other sicknesses.

C You lived in the city. You worked city jobs. You worked at docks. You worked in businesses with a lot of people. All of these put you at a higher risk for infection.

The plague infected all people. People could be healthy in the morning and dead by night.

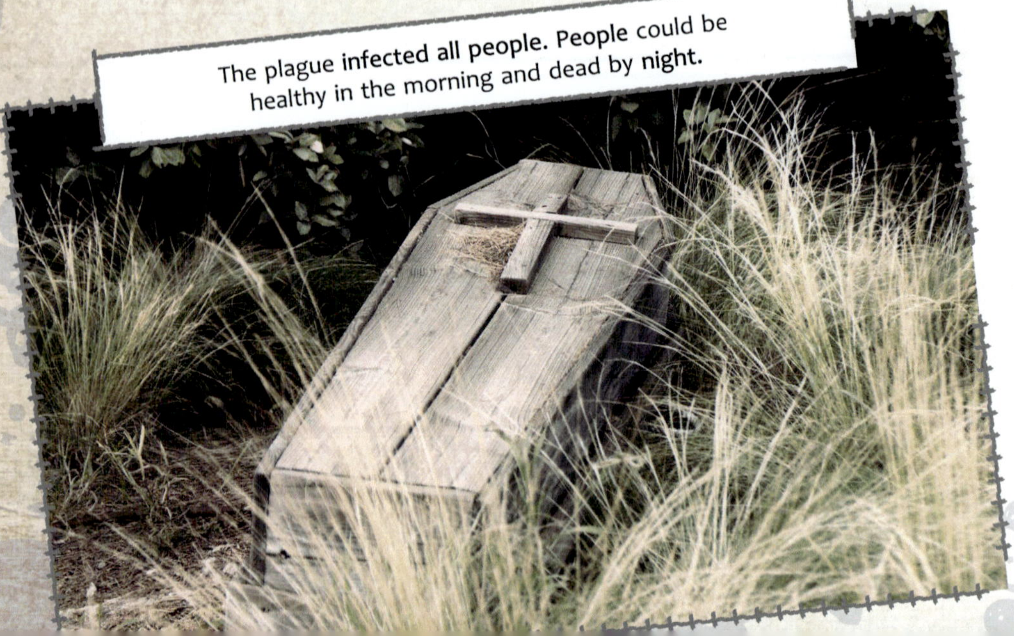

SURVIVOR BIOGRAPHY

Giovanni Boccaccio lived from 1313 to 1375. He was Italian. He was a writer and poet. He was from Florence, Italy. The plague killed about 75 percent of the people in Florence. He survived. He wrote about it. He wrote *The Decameron*. This book is a primary source about the plague. It's a collection of stories. It's about 10 people. There are 3 men and 7 women. They left Florence because of the plague. They escaped to the hills of Fiesole. They met for 10 days. They told each other stories. They did this to entertain themselves. The first chapter is about how the plague attacked Florence. Boccaccio describes how people felt. His book made readers feel better. It was a source of comfort. Boccaccio believed that love conquers all, even the Black Death.

STOP OR SPREAD?

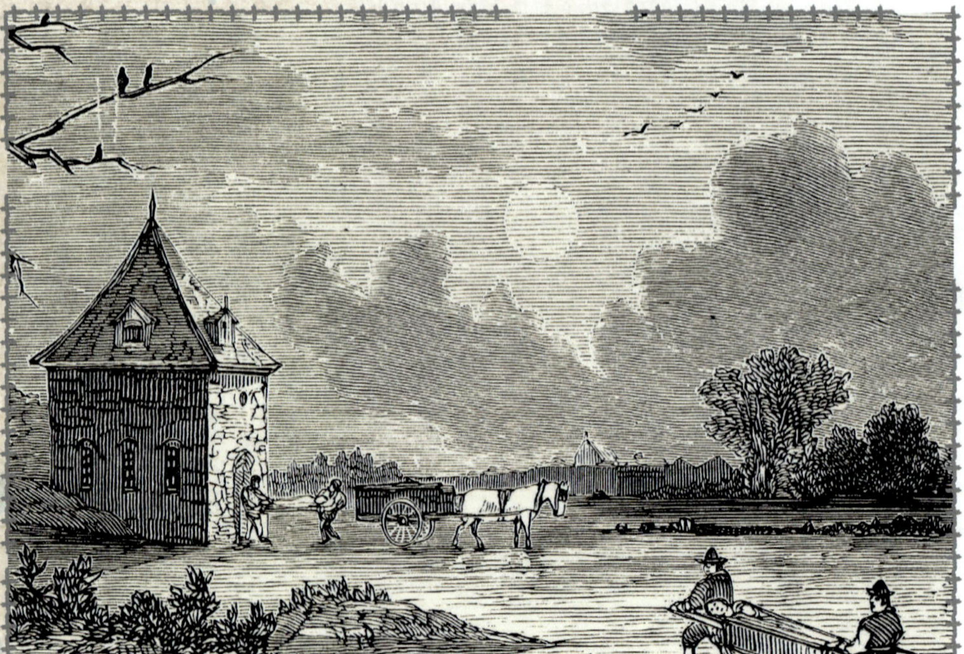

Quaranta giorni is Italian for "40 days." It's where the term quarantine comes from.

Venice is a city in Italy. During the Black Death, Venice officials organized the first plague response. Officials tried to stop the plague from spreading. They held sailors on ships for 40 days. They wouldn't let ships dock. This was called a **quarantine**.

Other cities organized public health actions. They inspected ships. They burned infected ships. They shut down restaurants. They banned food and wine from unknown sources. They made rules for how to take care of dead bodies.

Officials made infected people **isolate**. Isolate means to stay away from people. Officials wanted to make sure people didn't have any plague germs. Some cities created **lazarettos**. A lazaretto was an isolation hospital. Lazarettos were located far away from city centers but close enough to transport the sick.

QUESTION 2

What would you have done when you heard about the plague?

A You had enough money. You could afford not to work for a while. You isolated. You became a **recluse**. Recluses live apart from others.

B You were rich. You went to your country home. You quarantined with a few family members.

C You were poor. You had to continue to work. You had to go into the cities.

Infected people were quarantined in lazarettos.

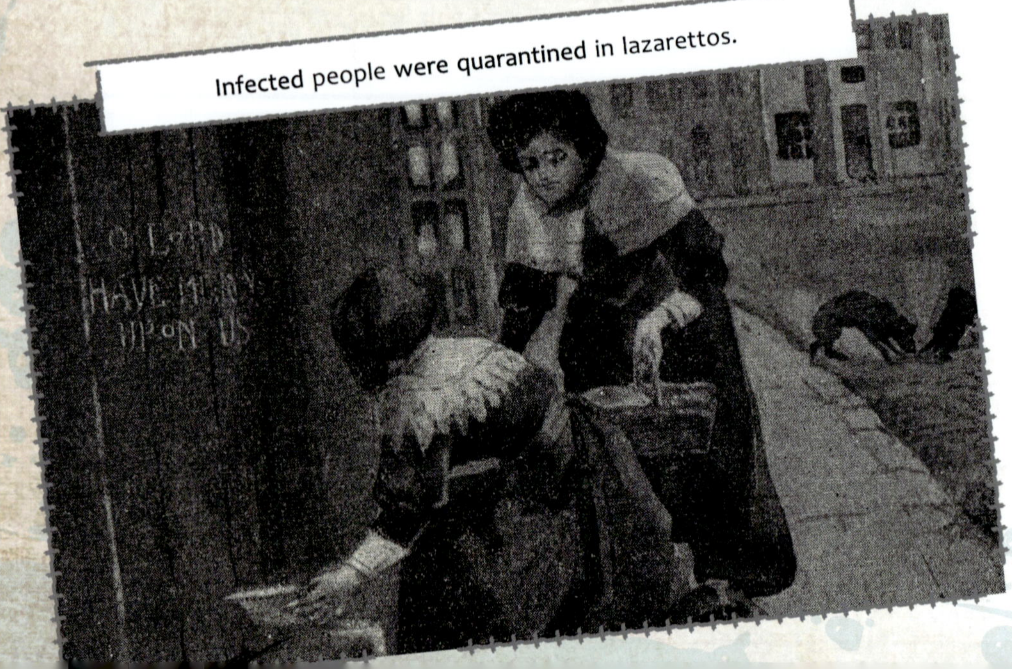

SURVIVAL BY THE NUMBERS

- The Black Death killed 75 million to 200 million people. This was 30 to 60 percent of Europe's people.
- In some villages, 80 to 90 percent of their populations died.
- The Black Death reduced the world's population in the 14th century from 475 million to 350 million people.
- At its worst, about 800 dead bodies were buried per day. On average, 20 to 60 bodies were buried daily. Many bodies were buried in the same pit.
- It took 300 to 400 years for population numbers to recover after the Black Death.
- The World Health Organization is in charge of public health. It states there are still 1,000 to 3,000 cases of plague every year.
- After infection, it takes 2 to 6 days for a bubonic plague victim to be sick.
- Without treatment, the bubonic plague kills up to 60 percent of victims.
- Over 80 percent of U.S. plague cases are bubonic plague. An average of 7 cases are reported per year.

SCIENCE OR SIN?

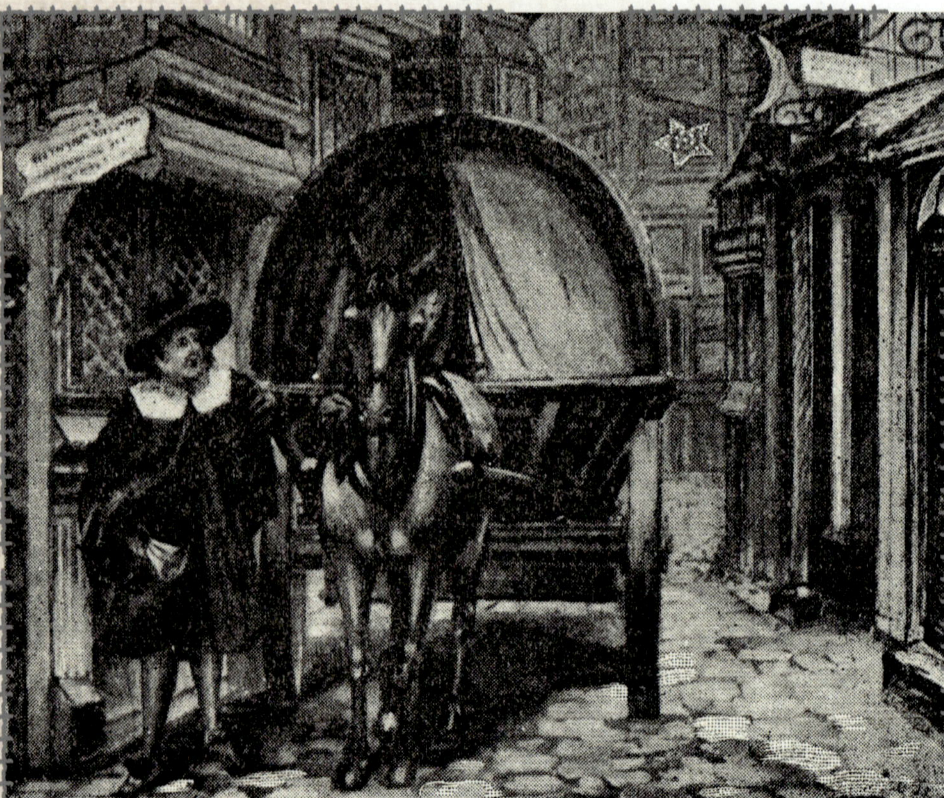

THE DEAD CART.

If one person was infected, everyone in the house would become infected as well.

In medieval England, people didn't understand the science of plagues.

Most Christian people thought the plague was a punishment from God. They thought they were being punished for their sins. They wanted to win God's forgiveness. They wanted to clean their souls. That's how they thought they'd stop the plague.

Some people purged their communities. They killed certain groups of people. They accused these people of being sinful.

Some people **flogged** themselves with heavy leather straps. Flog means to beat. These people joined groups of others doing this. They marched from town to town. This was a public display of **penance**. Penance is an act of self-harm to show devotion.

QUESTION 3

How religious were you during the plague?

A You weren't religious. You didn't know what caused the plague. But you knew to stay away from sick people.

B You were a practicing Christian. You prayed a lot. You wrote names of saints on paper. You put these papers on your body. You thought this kept away sickness and evil.

C You were a very religious upper-class man. You flogged yourself 3 times a day. You did this for 33 days.

Flogging put people at risk. Open cuts could become infected.

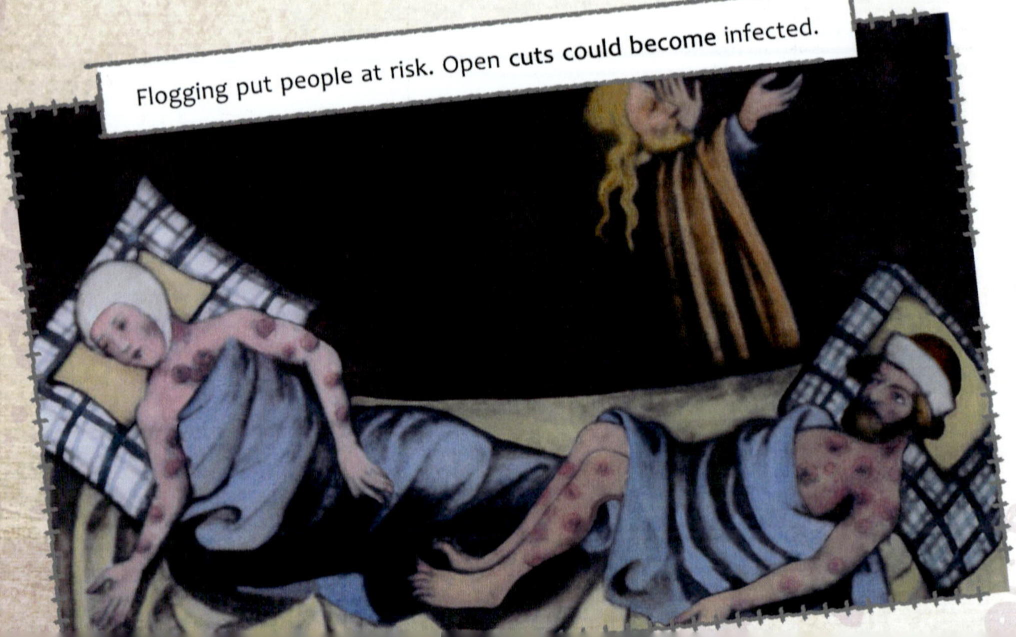

SURVIVAL TIPS

Follow these tips to survive the bubonic plague:

- Don't touch animals infected with plague germs.
- Stay away from sick and dead animals. Call your local animal control to pick them up.
- Avoid areas with wild rodents. Rodents include rats, squirrels, and chipmunks.
- Remove piles of leaves and sticks. Remove rock piles. Remove any areas that could attract rodents.
- Secure your trash. Keep wild animals away.
- Look for flea bites on your skin.
- Put flea collars on your pets.
- Don't let your pets roam free.
- Use bug spray to keep fleas away. Do this when camping or hiking.
- When you notice symptoms, get medicine from doctors. Do this within 24 hours of the first signs.

HEALER OR DOCTOR?

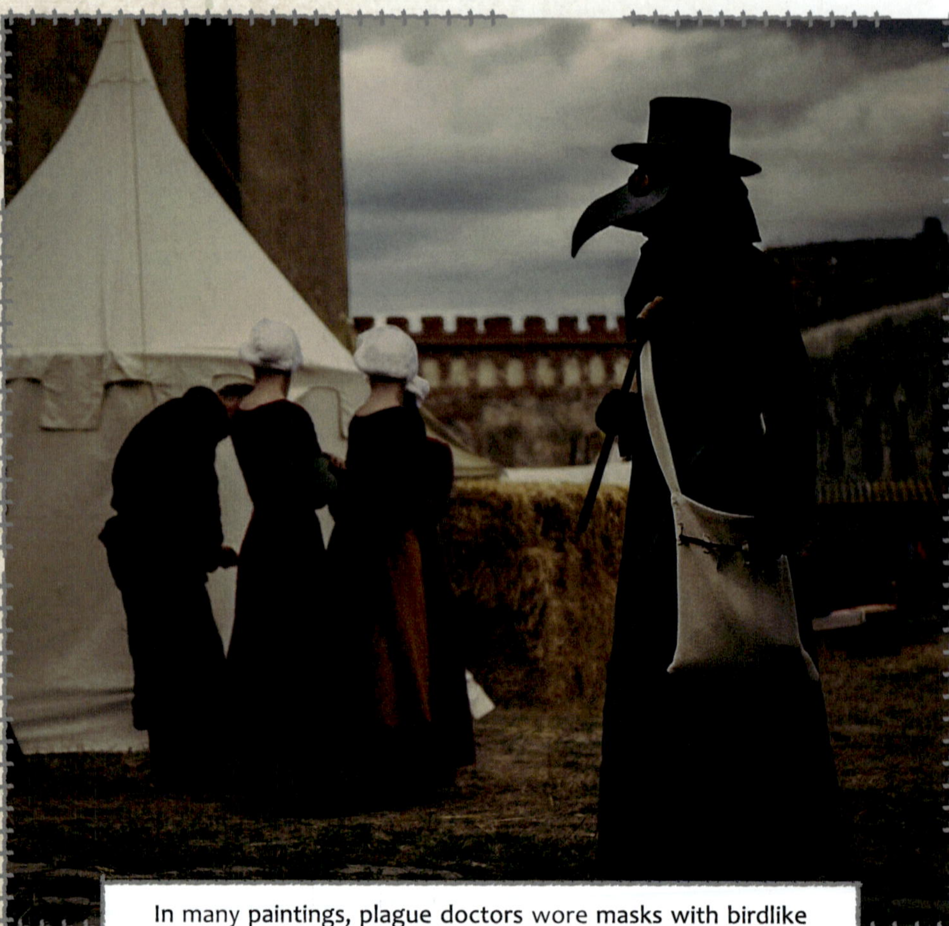

In many paintings, plague doctors wore masks with birdlike beaks. But the beak mask wasn't invented until 1619.

Medieval doctors didn't know much about the plague. They had two main treatment plans. One was **bloodletting**. Bloodletting is the removal of blood. Doctors wanted to get rid of bad blood. They wanted to rebalance the body. Plague doctors also **lanced** boils. Lance means to cut open.

Both bloodletting and lancing boils weren't effective. They didn't cure the plague. They were dangerous. They were **unsanitary**. Unsanitary is dirty.

People tried all kinds of things to cure the plague. Some people chopped up snakes. They put the snake bits on their boils. Some people drank the pus from boils. Some drank warm beer with eggshell bits. None of these things worked.

QUESTION 4

What type of medical help would you have gotten?

A You were working class. You went to a local healer. You were given herbal drinks. Healers knew about medicinal plants. They knew basic first aid. They didn't know how to cure the plague. But they knew how to help you feel less pain.

B You were rich. You could pay to see a doctor. Plague doctors would bleed you. They'd lance your boils. This could make you weaker.

C You were poor. You couldn't pay a doctor or healer. You practiced folk cures. These were not based on science.

Barbers cut hair. They also helped when needed as surgeons. They performed many operations in medieval Europe.

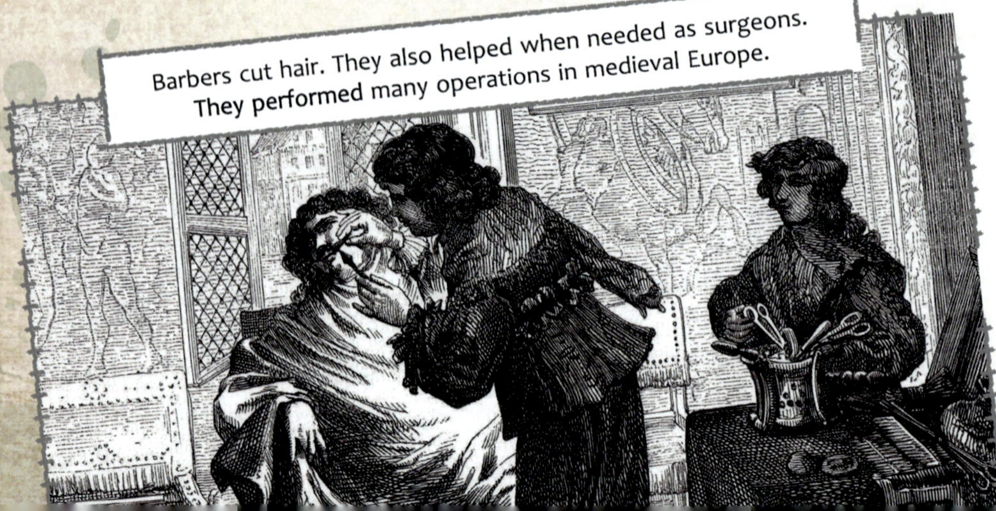

SURVIVAL TOOLS

Some people thought the plague was spread by bad air. Clearing the air was thought to be a cure. People in medieval England smoked out the air. They also carried flowers and herbs. They held these plants close to their faces. They stuffed plants up their noses. They put plants in their pockets. They put plants all around their houses. They did this to hide the smell of dead bodies. They thought this would clean their lungs. They also thought this would keep evil spirits away. The most popular flowers were roses. Rich people put roses in their water. They bathed in rosewater and vinegar. "Ring Around the Rosie" is a children's rhyme. Some people think this song is about the Black Death. "Rosie" refers to the red spots that turned black. "A pocketful of posies" refers to the flowers or herbs. The "ashes" refer to dead bodies. Dead bodies were burned. Victims' houses were burned.

THRIVE OR STARVE?

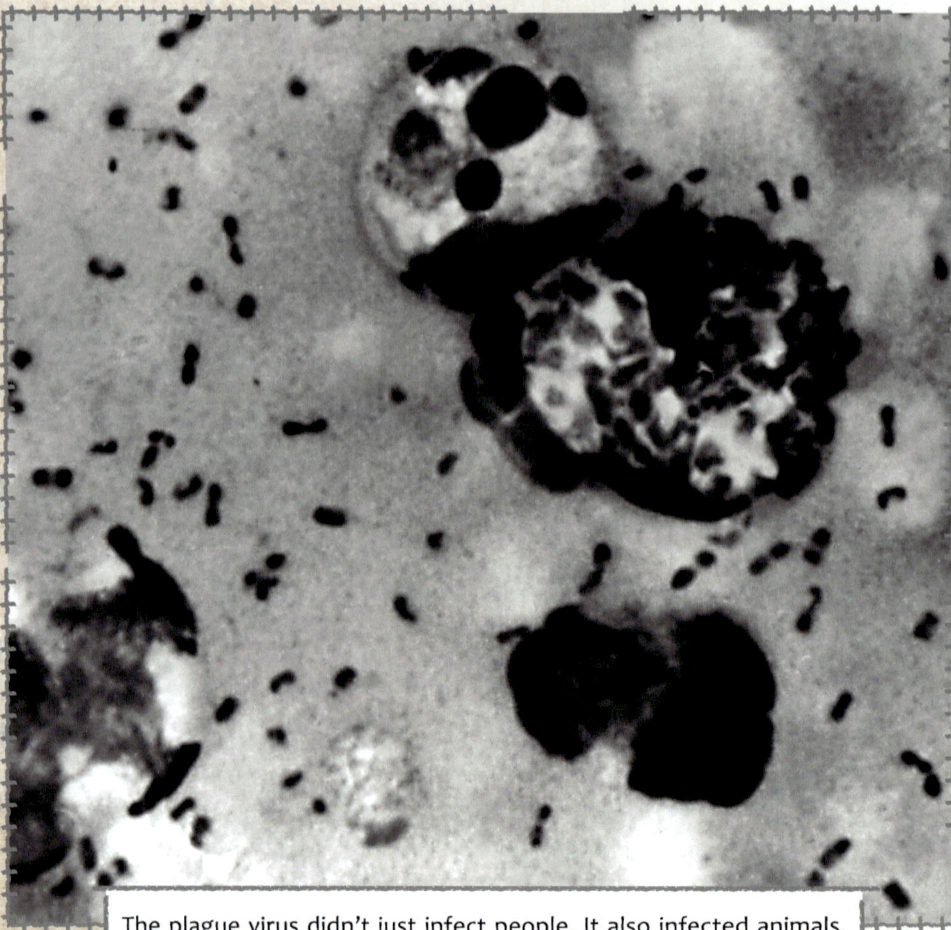

The plague virus didn't just infect people. It also infected animals.

The plague scared people. People didn't want to get sick. Doctors refused to see sick people. Store owners closed their shops. Family members left behind their sick loved ones.

People dying meant people weren't working. Businesses failed. Trade stopped. Nobody worked on farms. There was less food. People starved.

The plague also killed cows, goats, pigs, chickens, and sheep. Without sheep, there was no wool. There was a wool **shortage** in Europe. Shortage means a lack.

QUESTION 5

Would you have thrived during the plague?

A You were a church leader. People didn't know what was happening. They went to church for inner peace. They gave money. They gave their property. They wanted to secure their place in heaven.

B You were an **apothecary**. An apothecary sold medicines and drugs. People were desperate. They wanted to feel better. You made a lot of money selling "cures."

C You were a shopkeeper. You lost money. You lost your business. People weren't shopping. They were dead. They were poor. They were isolating.

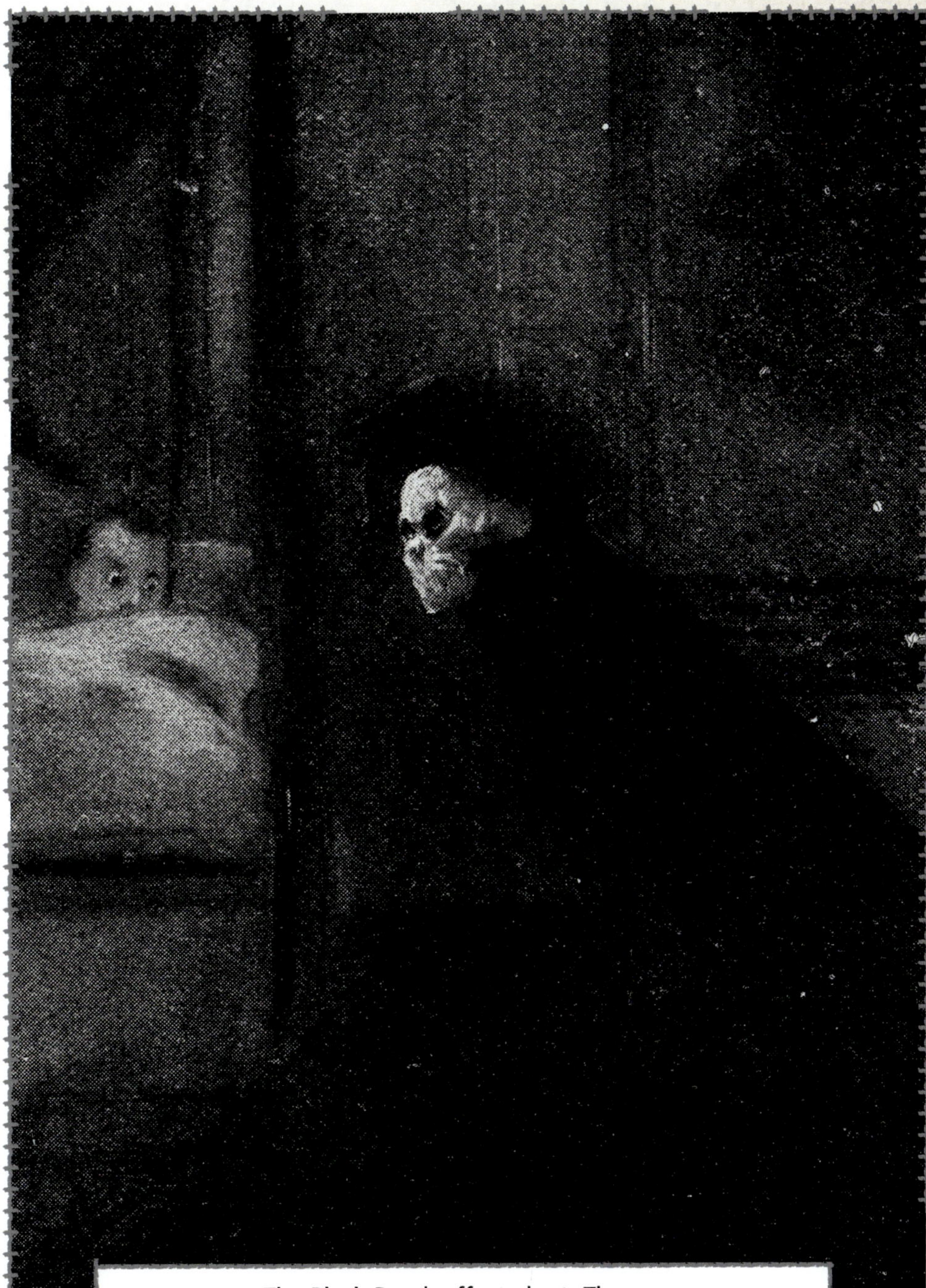

The Black Death affected art. Themes were dark and full of despair.

SURVIVAL RESULTS

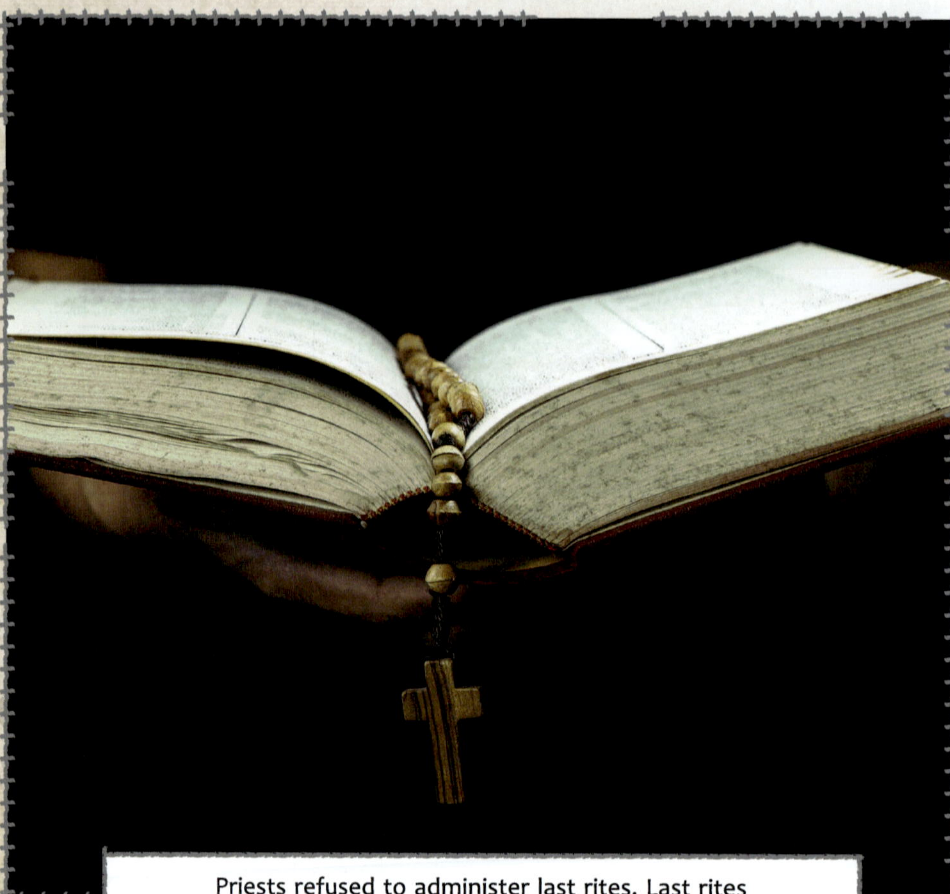

Priests refused to administer last rites. Last rites are prayers done shortly before death.

Would you have survived?

Find out! Add up your answers to the chapter questions. Did you have more **A**s, **B**s, or **C**s?

- If you had more **A**s, then you're a survivor! Congrats!
- If you had more **B**s, then you're on the edge. With some luck, you might have just made it.
- If you had more **C**s, then you wouldn't have survived.

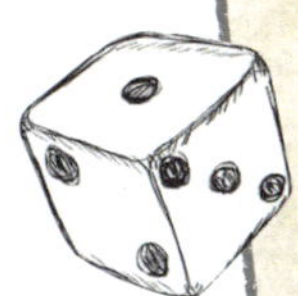

Are you happy with your results? Did you have a tie?

Sometimes fate is already decided for us. Follow the link below to our webpage. Scroll until you find the series name *Surviving History*. Click download. Print out the template. Follow the directions to create your own paper die. Read the book again. Roll the die to find your new answers. Did your fate change?

https://cherrylakepublishing.com/teaching_guides

DIGGING DEEPER: DID YOU KNOW ...?

The Black Death was a terrible time in history. Millions lost their lives. Surviving history involves many different factors. Dig deeper. Consider some of the facts below.

QUESTION 1:

How likely were you to get infected with the plague?

- Those who survived the plague had better chances of fighting future plagues.
- About 50 percent of plague cases occur in people ages 12 to 45.
- The plague infected more men than women.

QUESTION 2:

What would you have done when you heard about the plague?

- The number 40 had religious significance. It shows up often in the Christian Bible.
- Quarantine rules helped create a sense of order.
- The first lazaretto was located on an island in Venice.

QUESTION 3:

How religious were you during the plague?

- Medieval Christians were serious about their souls. They didn't want to go to hell.
- Saint Thomas Becket was a popular saint during the Black Death. People visited his shrine. Shrines are holy places.
- Men who flogged themselves in public were called **flagellants**.

QUESTION 4:

What type of medical help would you have gotten?

- Most healers were women. Most doctors were men.
- Some nuns learned medicine. They mainly delivered babies.
- Some people believed powder made from unicorn horns could cure them.

QUESTION 5:

Would you have thrived during the plague?

- There was a shortage of farmworkers. This meant landowners had to pay surviving workers more money.
- In England, over 1,300 villages were deserted between 1350 and 1500.
- Towns changed. People left. People died. People had to rebuild.

GLOSSARY

airborne (AIR-born) being able to be transported by air
apothecary (uh-PAH-thuh-kar-ee) a person who sells medicines and drugs
bloodletting (BLUHD-let-ing) a process of removing "bad blood" from the body
boils (BOILZ) bubbles on the skin
bubonic (boo-BAH-nik) caused by a swollen lymph node in the armpit or groin
flogged (FLAWGD) to beat oneself
infected (in-FEKT-id) made sick
isolate (EYE-suh-late) to keep away from others
lanced (LANTZD) cut open
lazarettos (lah-zur-ET-ohs) isolation hospitals
medieval (mee-DEE-vuhl) of the Middle Ages
pandemic (pan-DEM-ik) a sickness that spreads over a wide area
penance (PEH-nuhns) an act of self-harm to show devotion
plague (PLAYG) a sickness that spreads quickly
polluted (puh-LOOT-id) dirty
quarantine (KWOR-uhn-teen) holding infected people for a period of time in a place far from others
recluse (ruh-KLOOS) a person who lives apart from others
shortage (SHOR-tij) a lack or deficit
unsanitary (un-SAN-ih-ter-ee) dirty
victims (VIK-tuhmz) people who suffer

LEARN MORE!

- Griffin, Mary. *The Black Death.* New York, NY: Gareth Stevens Publishing, 2020.
- Jarrow, Gail. *Bubonic Panic: When Plague Invaded America.* Honesdale, PA: Calkins Creek, 2016.
- Krasner, Barbara. *Bubonic Plague: How the Black Death Changed History.* North Mankato, MN: Capstone Press, 2019.

INDEX

ABOUT THE AUTHOR

Dr. Virginia Loh-Hagan is an author, university professor, and former classroom teacher. She had to cancel a trip to Europe because of the COVID-19 pandemic. She lives in San Diego with her very tall husband and very naughty dogs.